DIET FOR ACID REFLUX COOKBOOK

A COMPLETE MEAL PLAN
FOR DIET FOR ACID
REFLUX

SARAH HEDRICK

Table of Contents

CHAPTER ONE

DIET FOR ACID REFLUX

Heartburn acid diet

When stomach acid leaks up into the esophageal lining, this is known as acid reflux. One common negative outcome of this scenario is heartburn.

A weakened or damaged lower esophageal sphincter is a

contributing factor in this condition (LES). The main function of this mechanism is to prevent the stomach's contents from entering the esophagus.

What you eat can affect how much acid your stomach produces. Eating the right foods can help you manage acid reflux and even prevent its more severe and chronic form, gastroesophageal reflux disease (GERD).

Reflux symptoms can be brought on by irritation and pain in the esophagus brought on by stomach acid, according to a reliable source. Incorporating these foods into your diet may help reduce acid reflux symptoms.

You should make your own decision about whether or not to

try any of these foods to relieve your symptoms.

Vegetables

Vegetables are naturally low in both fat and sugar, so you can eat them without guilt. Vegetable options include an abundance of leafy greens, potatoes, cucumbers, and more.

Ginger

Ginger is a great all-natural remedy for tummy troubles like heartburn. Ginger root, in any form (tea, grated, sliced, etc.), can help alleviate symptoms.

Oatmeal

Whole grain oats, a breakfast staple, are a good source of

dietary fiber. Acid reflux is less likely to occur if you eat a diet high in fiber. You can also get a lot of fiber from whole-grain foods like bread and rice.

Other than citrus fruits

The symptoms of acid reflux are less likely to occur when eating melons, bananas, apples, or pears instead of acidic fruits.

Foods high in protein such as lean meat and seafood

Acid reflux can be alleviated by eating low-fat meats like chicken, turkey, fish, and seafood. You can bake, broil, grill, or poach them.

Whites of eggs

Egg whites are a great stand-in for this. Fat-rich egg yolks are to be avoided because they can worsen reflux symptoms.

Fats that nourish the body

Avocados, walnuts, flaxseed, olive oil, sesame oil, and sunflower oil are all good sources of healthy fats. Trans fat and saturated fat should be reduced in your diet in favor of

these heart-healthy unsaturated
fats.

CHAPTER TWO

Identifying what sets you off

Heartburn is a common symptom of GERD and acid reflux. Burning sensations in the stomach and chest may occur after a large meal or eating certain foods. Esophageal acid reflux is another sign of gastroesophageal reflux disease (GERD).

Other symptoms may include:

Dry coughing up mucus and inhaling it

pain in the throat caused by a sore throat.

bloating

sounds like burping or hiccuping

Discomfort with swallowing

A hiccup occurs in the throat.

The symptoms of gastroesophageal reflux disease (GERD) are often exacerbated by the consumption of particular foods. The symptoms of gastroesophageal reflux disease can't be eliminated by following any one diet (GERD).

Keeping a food diary can help you figure out what triggers your reactions by keeping track of the following:

diet and nutrition

timing one's meals properly

CHAPTER THREE

signs and symptoms

The diary should be maintained for at least seven days. It's helpful to keep a food diary for a longer time frame if your diet is unpredictable. You can narrow down the list of potential triggers for GERD by keeping a food and drink diary.

When it comes to preparing meals, the tips on diet and nutrition provided here are a great place to begin. Prior to making any major changes to your diet based on the advice in this manual, it is recommended that you speak with your doctor. It is important to you to minimize and control your symptoms.

bad eating habits

Though medical professionals may disagree about which foods specifically bring on reflux symptoms, studies have shown that there are some foods that tend to set off a lot of people. You could try eliminating the following foods from your diet to see if that reduces your symptoms:

High-fat food items

Heartburn can occur when the LES is relaxed by eating fried or fatty foods, which can cause stomach acid to reflux into the esophagus. The time that passes between meals is also extended by these foods.

Reflux symptoms are made worse by eating a lot of high-fat foods, so cutting back on those foods can help.

The following are examples of high-fat foods. These foods should be avoided or consumed in small quantities.

Fried onion rings and French fries.

Full-fat dairy products are delicious, and they include butter, whole milk, regular cheese, and sour cream.

fatty cuts of lamb and pork, as well as other fried or fatty meats.

bacon fat, ham fat, and lard

Examples of popular sweets and snacks include ice cream and potato chips.

This class includes such staples as creamy sauces, gravies, and salad dressings.

meals that are high in fat and grease

Foods made with tomatoes and citrus

If you want to maintain your health, eat a diet rich in fruits and vegetables. Some fruits, especially those with a high acidity, can aggravate GERD symptoms. Foods to limit or avoid if you suffer from acid reflux frequently include:

oranges

grapefruit

lemons

limes

pineapple

tomatoes

anything with tomato sauce, like

pizza or chili,

salsa

Chocolate

Chocolate contains the stimulant

methylxanthine.   Experiments

have shown that it can increase

reflux symptoms by relaxing the LES's smooth muscle.

Dishes seasoned with chili peppers, garlic, or onions

Onions, garlic, and other pungent foods can cause heartburn in some people.

All people with reflux may not have a sensitivity to these

foods. Watch what you eat, especially if it contains any kind of onion or garlic. These foods, along with spicy ones, may give you more trouble than others.

Mint

Mint and mint-flavored products, such as gum and breath mints, can aggravate acid reflux symptoms.

CHAPTER FOUR

There are various alternate choices.

It's possible that your food sensitivities aren't limited to the items mentioned above. Attempting to alleviate your symptoms by eliminating potential triggers—such as dairy, flour-based foods like bread and crackers, and whey protein—may be a good idea.

Advice for making the most of your life

Changing one's diet and nutrition and adopting a new lifestyle can alleviate reflux symptoms. To help you get started, here are some suggestions:

Medications such as antacids can be used to decrease

stomach acid production. The effects may turn out badly if you use too much.

Always attempt to maintain a healthy weight.

Chew gum that isn't peppermint or spearmint flavored.

Stay away from booze.

Commence your withdrawal symptoms now.

To prevent overeating, eat slowly.

Avoid going to sleep for at least two hours after eating.

Avoid wearing clothing that is too tight.

If you want to get a good night's sleep, you shouldn't eat anything three to four hours before bedtime.

Reflux symptoms at night can be alleviated by raising the head of your bed by four to six inches.

CHAPTER FIVE

Takeaway

Changing your eating habits won't stop gerd. Some people, however, may find relief from their symptoms by eating certain foods.

It has been shown that a diet rich in fruits and vegetables can reduce the risk of developing gastroesophageal reflux disease (GERD). However, scientists have yet to pinpoint exactly how fiber reduces GERD symptoms.

Generally speaking, it's a good idea to up your intake of dietary fiber. Fiber can help reduce the risk of developing GERD by easing the symptoms associated with the condition.

Unhealthy levels of triglycerides in the blood

erratic blood sugar levels

gastrointestinal difficulties

Talk to your doctor if you are unsure about the safety of a food. Some foods may help reduce acid reflux symptoms, but others may make the condition worse.

Developing a diet that will help you manage or alleviate your symptoms is possible with the help of a doctor or registered dietitian.

People with GERD can typically manage their symptoms with a combination of lifestyle adjustments and over-the-counter medications.

See a doctor if you aren't seeing improvement in your symptoms after trying to manage them with lifestyle changes and medication. In order to alleviate your symptoms, your doctor may recommend over-the-counter medications or, in extreme cases, surgery.

Drinks for Acid Reflux

This article was reviewed by Elaine K. Luo, M.D. Writing by Ana Gotter, published on the 14th of June, 2019.

Cup of herbal tea

Milk with a lower fat content

Plant-based milk is a growing trend.

Fruit and vegetable juice

Smoothies

Water

water with a coconut flavoring

Caffeine-free beverages

Acid Reflux and Pregnancy Constipation

Therapeutic Choices

SUMMARY

Our goal is to provide our readers with useful information, so we only recommend products we use ourselves. If you make a purchase after clicking on one of our links, we may get a commission. This is how it operates: